Our Rightful Place in Health & Happiness

Healing Insights

SG Williams
BSc.(Hons) RAc.

ISBN: 978-1-7775584-0-6

DEDICATION

This world needs healing right now. There are many good souls out there spreading ripples of good energy everywhere they go. I know because I have been privileged to meet these wonderful people through my healing practice. This book was written for these beacons of light and for my husband Howard, who in every way, has been and continues to be, my earth angel.

CONTENTS

ACKNOWLEDGEMENTS

I thank my friends, my family and all the wonderful clients that I have had the pleasure of spending time with, over the past decade. Most of all, I thank my mother Marion and my husband Howard for their love, support and encouragement.

1 THE HEALING DILEMMA

Is there such a thing as good medicine? When I was young, medicine was always something that was good for you. Moms were always playing with their latest remedies like cod liver oil tablets or chew-able vitamins.

Then there is the everlasting search for miracle drugs. Remember the movie Medicine Man? The jungle was combed for an exotic flower with amazing cures. I loved that movie because of the scenery, Sean Connery, and because in those days, I was working in a pharmacology research lab. I was amazed how they could get that chromatograph to work in the jungle.

One of the pharmacology PhD students complained about a headache one day. When I offered Aspirin or Tylenol, she flatly refused saying, "I don't take any pills ever. You and I both know that there are bad side effects with every drug." She would know better than anyone else and so would I.

Drugs truly save lives and prolong life. I spent many years in pharmacology research. I believed in developing new and better drugs. I still do however drugs always have good wanted actions, bad unwanted side effects and if not taken in the proper therapeutic dosage range, for a specific situation, in the recommended conditions, either didn't work at all or were poisonous and lethal.

As years went by I wanted to be in a healing profession in a new way. As I prepared to apply to medical school, one of my children had bad migraines that nothing conventional was helping. Out of desperation, we tried acupuncture. It helped her. I tried it and it helped me. I then embarked on a quest to learn more and it changed my life.

I discovered, fell in love with and studied to become an acupuncturist. Acupuncture as practised within Traditional Chinese Medicine (TCM) is the good medicine I had been looking for. The results and side effects are always positive. Acupuncture fuels and facilitates our body's own natural healing abilities.

However, healing means different things to different people. Many believe that to be truly healed you need to address all levels of our being. Holistic healers and the traditional medicines actually link sickness to imbalances in the mind and physical manifestations of emotional dis-ease.

Holistic frameworks also attach our well-being to

the environment and our living conditions, our relationships and our social structures. Modern health promotion recognizes the tenets of health including things like social justice, housing availability as well as food scarcity.

Natural health stores have become much more mainstream as people accept the healing properties of plants that grow around us. There has been a resurgence of herbal medicine and this too is also one of the tools used in traditional holistic medicine.

There is also a very strong belief in the importance of good diet and exercise for optimum health. There is not always agreement of what form that should take. Many people have done their own research and have come to follow what they believe is healthy eating and good physical fitness.

Some ascribe to energy medicines and see the value of healing frequencies obtained through sound, touch and channeling. Positive thinking, meditation, visualization, laying on of hands, prayer as well as healing circles and pagan rituals, all fall within the world of healing.

There are tons of health gurus and healers to choose from. Each one may have ideas that can help us find our own way. Their prescriptions for health may not always meet all our unique needs or beliefs. After decades of study, observation and performing my own version of a healing practice, I started to see common patterns in all healing modalities practised by all the leading healers.

I believe that being happy and healthy are linked and that you can't have one without the other. Healing is a prerequisite for health and happiness. Good medicine recognizes our ability to heal ourselves and should not be complicated or expensive. I do not believe our creator would put us on this earth without the ability to do what we needed to thrive naturally and easily.

According to the Yellow Emperor's Classic of Medicine, there were four types of ancient peoples that existed on earth, a long time ago, that lived very long lives and did not display the usual signs of aging. The Immortals lived the longest, followed by the Sages, then the Achieved Beings and lastly the Naturalists who lived to over one hundred years.

The secret of their longevity was that they, "… lived simply…and close to nature…to prevent pathogens from invading." They got their energy from nature and lived in harmony with the environment, seasons, sun, moon and stars. They preserved their life force by adapting to society without adopting or getting pulled into popular thinking, cultural norms, emotional drama, excessive living, ambitions or desires.

These folks were able to heal themselves. When they got sick they "…guided properly the emotions and spirit and re-directed the energy flow…to heal the condition." If this did not work, they used herbs and herb-wines. Finally if a condition worsened, an accurate diagnosis with acupuncture and moxibustion, were used as an intervention to regain health and balance.

As a result of living simply, these folks also had remarkable abilities. They were able to travel freely outside the conventional view of time and space. They could see and hear far beyond what was considered normal. They were focused, accomplished much and kept a clear mind by integrating the mental, physical and spiritual with exercise, meditation, eating a balanced diet, at regular times and maintaining a pure conscience.

In Chinese medicine our life force, called Jing and health in general, is compromised by a weak constitution, emotional extremes, extremes in our external environment, overwork, inactivity as well as how, what and when we eat. This book, The Yellow Emperor, written approximately 2500 years ago, states "These days..." people's lifestyles have become detrimental to their health and they only live to fifty years or more. I believe this same statement is true today.

If we simplified our busy lives, got back to nature and focused more on what is most important to us, we would live longer and healthier lives. I am not so sure we would acquire supernatural abilities, but we would probably find more joy and happiness.

There are secrets to taking your rightful place in this world as the happy and healthy person you are meant to be. Alleviating dis-ease is all about raising your personal frequency and maintaining that vibration. It is not complicated but takes self examination and personal awareness. I can show you ways to affect the energy of your body, mind and spirit so you can be healed and heal others.

The cycle of the earth breathes the energy of birth, growth and decline. We too undergo a cycle of transformation that is beautiful and perfect.

Awaken to this rebirth and become aware of your magnificence. Love yourself wholly and accept the spirit of the universe that is at the core of who you are. Be in awe of every moment and see the magic in the ordinary. Cherish what you behold with new eyes.

Feel the peace of gratitude envelop you. Listen to your heart and seek your true self by dissolving the fog of the world. Be free. Know that you are perfect just as you are, wonderfully made and specially purposed.

Love the Earth. Embrace joy even in the most difficult times and know that you are loved, even if it is not a love from this world. Laugh, sing, dance and heal. Watch as your passions fulfill your deepest desires. Know that you can create the world of your dreams.
- SG Williams

2 TRY ACUPUNCTURE

My little ten pound min-pin, named Monster, looks up at me with such sad eyes and a forlorn expression. She is not the long legged little dog that you see in most of these breeds. She has short legs and a big belly and a stubborn, wilful attitude. I can almost hear her thoughts and I imagine her saying "Why would I let somebody, who is supposed to love me and take care of me, stick pins in me?"

She is right to ask that. We should all ask that same question because that somebody should not be just anybody who claims to do acupuncture. The profession is not regulated in our province. The amount of training varies greatly from certificates with hundreds of hours to full time, three year training, with over twenty-three hundred hours. The skill levels and types of disorders that can be successfully treated, varies dramatically.

Lucky for Monster, I am qualified. She soon found

out acupuncture is very safe when done by someone with adequate training. It does not hurt and can be very relaxing. Believe it or not, many of my clients think of my treatments as spa-like with the added health benefits. It will cause your body to correct any functions that may be a bit off. It will help heal anything that is injured and broken.

Even better, the World Health Organization did a comprehensive review of all the studies related to acupuncture, a number of years ago. They determined that acupuncture is safer than drugs when performed by a qualified practitioner. It was found that acupuncture boosts immunity, reduces pain, reduces inflammation and regulates body functions.

Acupuncture was determined to be effective for hundreds of conditions. Especially good, is that it can address chronic conditions. However acupuncture is just one tool used within a larger traditional holistic medicine framework that includes detailed diagnosis of patterns of imbalance, paired with lifestyle, herbs and other therapeutic modalities including nutrition and movement.

I mention acupuncture because it is a good way to regain our balance when we get lost. The Yellow Emperor's Classic of Medicine describes the practice of acupuncture still used by TCM acupuncturists today. I believe it was developed as an intervention, much like surgery is today, when people failed to live correctly and in tune with nature.

So while this ancient tool can get you back in the

game, it is not a replacement for self healing and maintaining good health. It is a good starting place if you are unwell and want to move forward on your path to wellness. That being said, it is pretty amazing when done right.

1. Acupuncture can help you feel that you can do anything.

2. Acupuncture can get you back to feeling your optimum self.

3. Acupuncture can help you feel more happy and calm.

4. Acupuncture helps awaken and energize our own self-healing capacity.

5. Acupuncture works, is safe and has no bad side effects.

6. Acupuncture will make you feel better and more balanced.

Acupuncture has been successful in helping with many ailments for thousands of years. Modern scientific data is being added to the body of evidence. Recent CT scanning has shown that unique areas on the body called acupuncture points do exist. Recently re-discovered staining techniques have uncovered a primo-vascular system that exists along acupuncture meridian pathways, where qi energy travels.

My little Monster had a bad cough for a few months

and became so weak, she could hardly walk. I gave
her two treatments of acupuncture. The next day she
was back to her old self. The results were dramatic. If
you believe that acupuncture only works because you
believe in it, then this is proof that it is not just a
placebo effect.

Acupuncture can get you moving in the right
direction but to stay in optimum health, you need to
get back to nature and listen to your body. It is
important to be with the people that support you. Seek
out work you are passionate about. Use the food and
herbs growing around you as medicine to keep you
strong. Think good thoughts, keep moving and be
grateful for everything. Just asking the universe will
help you discover your heart's desires.

*Medicine is not only a science; it is an art. It does
not consist of compounding oils and plasters; it deals
with the very processes of life, which must be
understood before they are guided...All that man
needs for health and healing has been provided by
God in nature, the challenge of science is to find it.*
- Paracelsus

3 Discover Herbs

I worked in science research for decades but I always wondered why the path to health and longevity was so expensive, technology dependent, difficult to achieve and in the hands of so few. Surely we came into existence with more accessible tools for health and survival? If the birds and little creatures in this world have everything they need to thrive, why not us?

I have a science background in agriculture and applied botany and I worked in pharmacology research for many years. I always believed however, that everything we needed to be healthy and all the tools we need to care for ourselves, should be readily available in nature. Early on I knew to use dandelion as a tonic in spring, coltsfoot for the lungs, plantain leaves for bleeding and chamomile for sleep. I had expected that western medicine could draw on the wisdom of plant medicine but that is not what I saw happening.

My first time in a pharmacy, when travelling in Europe, was a big surprise. Instead of rows of bottles, pills and supplements, I saw wall-to-wall shelves of dried herbs. It looked totally different than any pharmacy I had seen before. European pharmacies looked very much like many stores in the Chinatowns of our bigger cities, filled with dried herbs and formulas (combinations of herbs) for every ailment you could imagine.

Now that I am an acupuncturist and Chinese medicine practitioner, I have first hand knowledge of how to use and prescribe herbal medicine. My formulas have become invaluable to myself and many of my patients. They enhance and work hand in hand with acupuncture because of the common medical framework and diagnosis.

If you were diagnosed as having Liver Qi Stagnation, for example, there would be a specific point prescription that you could build based on the patient's underlying conditions. Then there would also be a matching herbal formula such as Xiao Yao San. I usually found that acupuncture was sufficient but stubborn or chronic conditions or cases where the patient was depleted, I found the herbal formulas were extremely beneficial.

I have a number of classic formulas that I rely on all the time. I use the classic formulas because they have been developed and used for thousands of years, have a wide range of herbs and therefore are well balanced, gentle and safe. Most of the herbal formulas depend on the skill of a qualified practitioner like myself, to ascertain a correct diagnosis before prescribing. Unlike acupuncture which is very forgiving, herbal medicine is not. The wrong formula can make a person's symptoms worse and the error may take days to resolve.

There are however some formulas that a lay person can use in moderation, by purchasing it themselves, over the counter. For example if someone has an upset stomach and diarrhea, Bao He Wan is a popular choice. For the first signs of an oncoming cold or flu where the throat is sore, I find that Yin Chiao is excellent. It will stop the virus from developing further if caught soon enough. I keep this on hand for a possible Covid19 exposure. I believe it will reduce the effects if I get it.

For infections especially for the chest, I use Andrographis. It is a powerful antibiotic and antiviral. For injuries like sprains, to accelerate healing and reduce swelling, Zheng Gu Shui should be a go to. For chronic pain conditions that are not from deep seated conditions like a hip disorder, I use That Stuff for Pain. It is an all natural product made in Canada. For some things it is all you need. For deep seated chronic pain, it can help reduce the reliance on more harmful pills and painkillers.

The number of Chinese formulas is extensive. There are many large volumes of ancient Materia Medica available that you could spend years perusing. Each formula is well balanced and draws on the healing abilities, properties and synergies of a number of plants. Many of these plants have never been heard of in the west. My shelves are lined with largely unknown, natural antivirals, antibiotics, painkillers, immune boosters, digestive strengtheners, cholesterol reducers, cough suppressants, menstrual regulators, diuretics, anti-allergenic, anti-diarrhea formulas, fertility boosters, blood builders, energy boosters, calming herbs to regulate anxiety and herbs to improve and combat vision loss, to name many but not all of them.

Western drug companies are now investigating Chinese herbs because they have healing benefits and treat conditions that have no cures in western medicine. The herbal companies in China continue to grow and become better regulated in terms of quality. I get my herbs from a company in New Mexico that oversees quality production in Taiwan. Well-respected doctors in my field endorse the products. I always know I am getting a quality product that is the same every time.

China's traditional medicine, that includes acupuncture and herbs, is regarded as a national treasure and is exported around the world. They integrated their thousand-year-old traditions with modern medicine. I believe it was partly because it was the only affordable way to treat such a large population of people. At a hospital in China you will have your modern MRI and surgery in the same place as your herbal medicine, acupuncture and qigong.

We have a strong western herbal tradition here in North America and many health food stores now carry herbal remedies based on this tradition. Our own natural food and supplement stores are growing in popularity. We too have a national treasure that needs to be developed further for a healthier, sustainable and affordable way to keep ourselves well. We have a number of knowledgeable herbalists. It is always best to consult a qualified herbalist even though some of the specialty stores have someone to help you select the right herbs.

I believe that for every illness or ailment known to man, that God has a plant out here that will heal it. We just need to keep discovering the properties for natural healing.
- Vannoy Gentles Fite

...

The art of healing comes from nature, not from the physician. Therefore the physician must start from nature with an open mind...
- Paracelsus

4 LIVE BY THE SEASONS

Spring Has Sprung, But Have You!

Spring is the time of the wood element. This element corresponds to the liver and gallbladder, the direction is east, the manifestation is wind, the colour green and the taste is sour. In us, wood controls the sinews and tendons, opens into the eyes, manifests in the nails and in the emotion of anger.

For all of us the excitement mounts as the weather gets warmer and we can look forward to getting outside more. People who are constitutionally wood types, like to be busy and will be especially anxious to break free of the confines of the winter cocoon to pioneer their new adventures. These folks will have well developed plans and be focused.

To be your optimum self, the yin and yang in us must be balanced. Any deficiencies or excesses create a pattern of imbalance that affects our qi, our body fluids and the function of our organs that are represented by the elements. As in the world around you, the elements have relationships that follow rules of order. So too do our organs and body functions have relationships and work together according to particular frameworks and rules. When upset, changes show up as imbalances in our body, mind and spirit. In TCM we have a number of medical frameworks outlining the rules that help us diagnose the problem in the relationship within the body that caused the symptoms.

If your wood element is well balanced, you will feel supple, resilient and be able to move and bend like a tree when the winds of change blow. You will have a clear vision of your plans, what you are doing, what you want to accomplish and why. You will have energy, will power and the information you need to make decisions. Determination will be in your circle of friends. No obstacle will be able to stop your creativity as you find alternative ways to reach your goals, if needed.

If you have a significant imbalance affecting your wood element, you may be suffering one or more issues like headaches, red, itchy or watery eyes, stiff tendons, bizarre dreams and reproductive or menstrual issues like PMS (premenstrual syndrome). Mentally, you may lose motivation, feel stuck, lose sight of your vision (your plan and your sight). Emotionally, you may feel irritable or even have outbursts of anger when the imbalance is rooted in the liver. If it is the gallbladder that is affected, you may feel more timid than usual and be plagued by indecision.

Spring is the time we are supposed to burst forth with renewed energy but we need to look to nature for our queues. During the long winter we were meant to rest and recharge our resources. If we did not do that well, like spending inordinate amounts of time shovelling snow (my personal experience), we may want to rest a bit longer. It would be prudent to gather more energy before tackling any big projects this season.

This is not an issue because spring is moving very slowly on the eastern shore of our province. It is now the middle of May, the mayflowers have just recently bloomed and the buds on the trees have only now slowly transformed into little leaflets. Even the crocuses are behind schedule compared to the rest of the world.

Springtime can be windy with the cold breezes still briskly moving from the north toward the eastern shores of the ocean. Wind is an issue for this season so it is important to continue to dress warm and keep your neck covered with a scarf. Hold off on the cold salads, cool drinks and fast cooked foods. Continue to nourish yourself with immune boosting herbs (astragalus or ginseng for example) and slow cooked soups (with warming herbs such as ginger and garlic) and stews (with antivirals like rosemary, sage or thyme) until you feel ready.

Summer Time, the Happy Season!

Summer is the time of the fire element and is about the heart, relationships, joy, laughter and heat. This can translate to passion and a focus on intimate relationships as well as lots of socializing and partying within the wider scope of friendship. The heart helps us be our true self and works with our intuition. This element is paired with the small intestine which represents clarity, discernment and judgment needed to see what is good for us and who is not.

The heart opens to the tongue, shows up in the complexion and is responsible for the blood. It is also the house of the Shen (ruler of the mind, emotions and thought). You can observe it when you look into someone's eyes. If it is good, the eyes are bright, clear and the person is appropriately engaged in your conversation.

Excellent Shen manifests as sparkling eyes. People with this recover well from any illness, no matter how severe. Poor Shen shows itself when the person cannot look you in the eye or you get the feeling the person is not truly present, that nobody is home. This happens to many people who have experienced trauma or abuse. It is a protective mechanism. These folks may not heal as quickly as others.

A person who is predominantly a fire element in their constitutional makeup, can have a singing voice, is often charming, the life of the party and likes to socialize and stay connected to others. When the heart is not in balance, the opposite happens and the person does not feel like talking to others and at the severe end of the spectrum, may have difficulty speaking. Mentally and emotionally a person may experience mood swings, dream disturbed sleep or possible heart palpitations or chest oppression.

The taste of summer is burnt which coincides with the barbecue season. Summer is the time for doing, going to parties, having fun and roasting stuff. Meals should be lightly cooked with steam or simmering, high heat and short cooking times. Foods for summer include alfalfa, apples, cucumber, watermelon, bitter greens like dandelion as well as Swiss chard, romaine, broccoli, celery.

Summer is the time to take an adventure and have fun. Joy is the emotion of this element. Be active, visit friends and family and laugh a lot. The water element controls fire and will help you stay balanced. The fluid associated with the fire element is sweat, so drink lots of liquids (cool is OK and add a pinch of salt and sugar for the electrolytes). The peak time for the heart is eleven in the morning until one in the afternoon, so be active morning to midday and rest in the afternoon. Remember that summer is the season of fire and that could also translate to burn-out.

Late Summer, Earth Time!

Late summer is the time of year where the shadows grow longer and we notice the freshness of the air at dawn and dusk. This is the descent into fall-autumn where the glory of the summer warmth hangs suspended in our memories. Late summer is the peak time of the earth element when the colours of the landscape show up in many variations of yellow (the colour of earth) and the harvest is ready.

Late summer is also a time of peace and of abundance. Just as the dense earth nourishes and roots the trees, so too do the organs of this element, the spleen and stomach, nourish and root us. These organs are the earth element in us and they are responsible for transforming and transporting our food to nourish us with post-heavenly qi.

People with a predominantly earth archetype are the peacemakers and those we call the salt of the earth. These are the people that establish, sustain and nurture relationships. They are those people in our lives that keep families and communities together. They are sensitive and reactive to the needs of others and embody sympathy, caring and friendship. The earth is our centre of gravity in both our interior and exterior, that allows us to move and change through life without losing balance.

This is the time of year that we will have more issues with our spleen or stomach and it becomes easier for the earth in us to become unbalanced. Paired with the position of the stars right now, the tensions in the world and the pandemic, we will need to watch how, what and when we eat to keep emotions of worry, obsessive thinking and self-doubt in check. The power of earth comes from the ability to link up with others and sustain a good balance between personal relationships, alone time and building community.

Autumn, Time to Reflect

Fall-autumn is the time of year for the metal element where we witness nature at its most brilliant self. The trees let go of their colourful mantle and the water takes on the sheen of mercury as it becomes still and cold. The weather alternates between cool and warm with a freshness in the air at dawn and dusk. The wind alternates between calm and increased breeze as its direction shifts from south-west to north-east signifying change is upon us.

The metal element governs our skin, nose, water passages, mucous membranes, respiration and the strength of our voice. The organ systems that correspond to this element are the lung and large intestine. These represent what comes into our lives and what needs to be eliminated. The emotion is grief. Just as the trees let go of their leaves, so we too need to acknowledge our losses and let them go as we prepare for a new chapter in our lives.

Now is the time to be mindful, reflect on our blessings and take an inventory of everything we have accomplished. Just like the phases of the moon from new to full, the plants of the earth have bloomed and produced its fruit. Everything has come to fruition. Like the trees that have shed their leaves, we too have the opportunity to shed the things that no longer serve us well. That gives us room for change.

People with a predominantly metal archetype like order and value the finer things in life. They like rules, simplicity and find inspiration in what is right.

They are guided by courage and the conviction of their principles. The colour of this element is white and represents purity. The lung rules the wei qi. This is the defensive energy that protects us at the skin level. The metal people in our lives also protect us and watch over us and keep us on the straight and narrow path.

So as the days get shorter, we will need to pay more attention to what we eat, what we wear and what we think, paying special attention to our mental health. This season can bring more lung issues and we can become pensive, worried or sad. Now is the time to eat pungent, savoury, spicy and warming foods, nutritious soups, stews, herbs to boost immunity, don socks and scarves to keep us warm and stay positive. It helps to be grateful for everything no matter how small.

Winter, Time for Regeneration

The air is so fresh and clean this time of year. Summer and fall are loud months. Soon we will enjoy the silence as people move indoors and the falling snow acts as a buffer that insulates and deadens the noise. That leaves us time to think. If you are constitutionally a water type (the winter element is water), you will look forward to the quiet, slower pace.

The snow protects gardens and plants from extreme temperature fluctuations, provides needed moisture and nourishes the soil with nitrogen from the atmosphere. It also insulates many small creatures and hides their food stores. Look carefully after a fresh snow and you will see many tracks left by wildlife that you may not even know live around you.

Winter is the time for contemplation, introspection, hibernating, conserving energy and going inward. We can think about what we are doing to connect with our passions and dreams. This is the real beginning of the year. The pure white landscape and sparkle of sunlight reflecting off the snow, reminds us of purity and gives us a blank canvas for a fresh start.

The winter water element is represented in the colours of dark blue and black. The emotion is fear but is also connected to willpower, hope and potential. The sound is groaning and the organs are the kidneys and the bladder. The kidneys open to the ears, support the bones, influence hair growth and lays the foundations for fertility.

The Ming Men are located between and near the kidneys. It stores our prenatal life force called Jing or pre-heaven qi. As we work our way through life, this qi gets depleted. When it is gone, so are we. However, we can preserve this life force by living well and increasing our post-heavenly qi. This is the qi we get by eating good food we obtain through the air we breathe and food we eat. Winter is the most important time to slow down and regenerate so we can protect this life force.

Now is not the time for strenuous exercise, fasting and cleansing diets. In fact it is OK to put on a few extra pounds. Salty and bitter flavours support the kidneys and they promote a sinking, centring quality that helps our kidney Qi. Foods such as miso, seaweed and soya sauce combined with bitter turnip are good in stews with warming black pepper, cinnamon and onion. Warming proteins like egg, black bean and pork, slow cooked at low temperature are ideal. Especially beneficial is any soup made with bone broth.

While you practice patience in this quiet time, pamper yourself with healing sounds, pure essential oils and a good book, while keeping your neck, feet and lower back warm to prevent the cold and damp from settling in. The ancient sages tell us to live in harmony with nature and the patterns of the seasons. Therefore it is appropriate to go to bed early and sleep in. Turn the lights down in the evening, light some candles then curl up by a heat source and take time to rejuvenate your whole self in body, mind and spirit.

*Man is a microcosm, or a little world, because he
is an extract from all the stars and planets of the
whole firmament, from the earth and the elements;
and so he is their quintessence.*
- Paracelsus

5 USE FOOD AS MEDICINE

What to Eat? Looking Back for Perspective

There is so much confusion and conflicting reports about what we need to eat to be healthy, that many people are saying, "I don't know what to eat anymore." My thought is that surely someone smart enough to put the human race on this planet, would be smart enough to give us the resources to survive and thrive.

The discussion about the latest and greatest super food and arch villain of the edible world, is almost as popular as the weather. Almost everyone talks about it and people have become very polarized in their beliefs about food. What to eat and what you believe about nutrition runs as deep and is just as sensitive as talking about religion, in some circles.

The answer lies in looking to our past. Our ancestors grew their own food, ate the animals they raised or hunted and lived off the land. According to studies looking back at all the historical data, our parents, parents, parents, did not have the same levels of health issues we have today with diabetes, obesity, infertility, heart disease, autoimmune disorders, depression, anxiety etc. Also they did not have shorter life spans, as some people would have us believe.

According to some emerging and controversial experts, we are essentially malnourished because of what we eat in our modern diets. There is much science looking back at large amounts of data and trends pointing to the importance of the traditional diet. This makes so much sense to me and I believe this is the common sense we forgot. Every food below under Do Eat contains vital substances that our bodies need to grow, develop, repair and thrive.

Here is a summary of what I am learning about our traditional diets that we need to adopt to be healthy. If you have heard older folks say, eat everything in moderation, I too ascribe to this and recommend it. This sums up some of what I believe we should eat.

Do Eat:
Fermented foods like sauerkraut, kimchi, yogurt, kombucha, pickles (no vinegar), seaweed, organ meats, grass fed beef, free range eggs, cod liver oil, fish eggs, fish such as salmon or herring, lots of vegetables cooked with a little fat, cooked green vegetables, kale, broccoli, cauliflower, turnip, onion family vegetables like leeks, onions, mushrooms especially those growing on trees like chaga, brightly coloured vegetables, soup stocks especially like bone

broth, whole milk, butter, lard, bacon fat, coconut oil, pure olive oil, fruits in season like berries. Variety is important. Make sure to eat as many food groups as possible. The food source is also key. Eat real, whole, fresh, natural food found as close to the source as possible, i.e. local.

Do Not Eat or Eat with Caution:

Sugar, carbohydrates, artificial sweeteners, grains, nuts, and seeds unless they are sprouted, processed oils, fats that are low quality, processed foods, soda drinks, distilled water and soy products. Do not remove fat. Do not remove any specific food group. Avoid restrictive diets.

It is Not Just about What you Eat

Did you know that the nature or properties of the foods you eat, how you eat and your frame of mind, affects nutritional intake and ultimate wellness?

The stomach and spleen are paired in our TCM framework. Together these organs, along with the lung and small intestine system, provides the life-giving energy the body needs to feed and protect itself. Many imbalances and health issues according to TCM diagnosis, start with stomach and spleen issues. The spleen and stomach as well as the lung also play a large role in immunity in our traditional medicine. Western medical practitioners and naturopaths also believe many problems related to health, such as inflammation, allergies and autoimmune disorders, start with digestive problems.

According to TCM, the stomach and spleen are responsible for transformation and transportation of nutrients and fluids. The stomach likes dampness, warm temperatures and is affected by emotions. The stomach and spleen dominate muscle strength, control blood and transform dampness. Examples of symptoms related to issues with the spleen and stomach show up as pale colouring to the lips, yellowing of complexion and around the mouth, fatigue, diarrhea, easy bruising, prolapses, varicose veins, edema, nausea, digestive issues (bloating, gas, pain), lack of taste, heavy limbs and prolonged and irregular menstruation or bleeding.

The nature of the food is important. Overly spicy

food or dry food can aggravate the stomach causing heat or yin deficiency problems. Cold or raw foods can cause stagnation with bloating, gas, flatulence or pain. If you already have a cold imbalance then it is OK to eat spicy foods. If you already have a heat imbalance then cold and raw is OK. The situation is different for every person. If you find you are ravenous for food at certain times of the day, chances are you have stomach heat. Food consisting of a warm, moist, neutral balance is best.

In terms of how you eat, it is important to chew well and eat meals at regular times. Don't over-indulge, eat too fast, nibble, read while eating, eat too late at night, think about work, worry, or be sad or angry while eating. Emotional strain is a detriment to good digestion. A positive frame of mind is best. In particular, worrying, over thinking and over analyzing, even when not eating, can affect digestion over a long period of time and can lead to chronic deficiencies.

So my advice is to be mindful of your eating habits, maintain a balance of temperature and moisture, chew well, eat on a regular schedule and be happy when eating! Most of all be grateful for the food and all the plants and animals that nourish you. They are gifts from the universe.

Be kind to yourself. Forgive your own imperfections. You are uniquely made. You have a special destiny. Reflect on the good in you. Accept the many facets of love. It is time to receive and be grateful for the gifts the universe has made for you. -SG Williams

42

To Mow or Not to Mow, That is the Question

Today while mowing my lawn, I became increasingly uncomfortable as I saw how I was decapitating the tops of the lovely little chickweed flowers, bluets, purple self-heal, tall yellow hawkweed, violets, wood sorrel and other unnamed little plants that I have yet to identify. My lawn is really a closet meadow, very little actual grass. I was mowing because I was caving to the expectation that my lawn be green, neat and short.

Conformity, sameness and bland is what the world expects, wants and is comfortable with. The trend in the populated areas is houses on streets with restrictive covenants to ensure some level of sameness. Gardens organized and planned to have colour splashes, height and textures in just the right spots. Lawns that are uniform green and weeded, so only the chosen plants grow.

Then I thought about what I love about my home and why I want to be here. Each of us has carved out our own unique, unconventional homesteads dotted in every nook and cranny along the shore. I love our collection of non-matching homes, yard structures, escaped gardens, wild roses on the sides of the roads, chicken coops, sheds of all kinds, garages without a roof, beached boats and old cars in fields on blocks.

People from the city are sometimes uncomfortable at first as they travel along our roads. They find it unsettling to see big houses, small ones, bright and many colours, additions in odd configurations, lavish and humble, all mixed together. Could this randomness be a reflection of who we are, rebels against conformity?

Did you know that a small drop of water in a lupin leaf looks exactly like a diamond? This small gem would have gone unnoticed if I had not been paying attention and asked my husband to take a picture of it. I almost missed it. Nature in all its randomness is so much more beautiful than any landscape or structure we try to create.

So I have come to a decision. I don't have to mow if I don't want to. I am vowing to not mow again this season. Sorry neighbours, but I have a whole meadow of healing herbs that I want to explore before the summer is over.

Now as the years have passed, my yard has become a medicine chest. These weeds are food with rich nutrients and properties that I can use to enhance my everyday meals. Heal-all is called that for a reason. I have chaga growing on an old birch tree right across from my clinic door. Eyebright is an endangered plant and grows profusely in the wild areas I purposely no longer tend or manage.

So as I am writing this, I am making my own bone broth that I fortify with Chinese herbs such as astragalus, licorice root, jujube dates, goji berries, reishi mushroom, shiitake mushroom and plants from my own yard. I also add the aromatic herbs of sage, rosemary, thyme, oregano and parsley that I grow in my garden, plus fresh garlic, ginger and onion. The resulting broth is used as a basis for soups and stews or for cooking rice.

The soil I use for my gardens is almost exclusively made from the material I composted in the previous year. I add compostable cat litter after the non-urine parts are removed. Ashes from my wood stove are used to sweeten the lawn and wild areas, put back nutrients and raise the pH to improve absorption. This way not only can I fortify my diet with the plants the universe has provided me with, I can be sure that both my wild and cultivated plants are happy and nutritious.

6 KEEP MOVING

If you don't move, you will lose muscle mass, put on weight and lack energy. The qi in the body needs to flow. When it is not flowing properly, the result is pain, dysfunction and symptoms of imbalances. In order for it to flow there needs to be enough fluid, blood and yin that is acquired by living properly and eating right.

Lack of movement can cause all kinds of obstructions like cold and damp conditions that can cause the clear rivers of Qi to behave more like muddy puddles. When there is no movement of qi there are deficiencies that can cause fatigue and failure to transform and transmute fluids properly. This can cause weight gain, digestive issues, water retention, swelling and more.

Unless you are trying to increase endurance or strength for a particular purpose, you don't need to run a marathon or work out in the gym. Walking at a good pace in the fresh air is perfect. Ideally you want to do at least twenty or thirty minutes a day. Wear comfortable shoes and if you can walk in nature, looking at the trees and breathing in the oxygen the trees put out, have extra benefits of helping you feel calmer and more grounded.

Learn Qigong

Qigong is an ancient Chinese therapeutic movement that looks a bit like Tai Chi but concentrates on the medical aspects of health and supporting body systems. "Qi" stands for the qi energy that is being cultivated and "Gong" means mastery. It is beautifully gentle and for all ages. It also teaches breathing, visualization and how to increase your qi. It can be combined with mediation and is easy to build into a daily routine as it can be done anywhere.

Qigong is key to a holistic practice in TCM and is taught along with acupuncture, herbal medicine and other tools for improving health like Tui Na which is a form of massage. Between treatments of acupuncture and along with herbal formulas, qigong is also recommended and often prescribed. The guided movements and controlled breathing are designed to keep specific meridian channels open and clear. It can also include self massage, sound and focused intent.

Many have found that this particular practice can help improve the immune system, reduce stress and help with focus and balance. The movements facilitate a more balanced body in terms of function, by resetting the body to neutral and releasing blockages in the energy flow. My favourite set of movements is called the Eight Brocade because it is comprehensive and easy to remember. There are many examples of this on the internet if you look at YouTube.

Qi(chi) is the Chinese term for life energy, or life

spirit, a vital force that flows through all living things. It is an essential part of Traditional Chinese Medicine, acupuncture, qigong and the Chinese martial arts. When our Qi is in harmony, we tend towards wellness, health and longevity. When our Qi is in disharmony we tend towards disease, suffering and collapse.
- Subtle Energy Sciences

...

When you cultivate balance and harmony within yourself, or in the world, that is Tai Chi. When you work and play with the essence of energy of life, nature and the universe for healing, clarity and inner peace, this is Qigong.
- Roger Jahnke

7 ENHANCE YOUR ENVIRONMENT

*You are a product of your environment, so choose the
environment that will develop you towards your
objective. Analyze your life in terms of your
environment. Are the things around you helping you
toward success or are they holding you back?*
- W. Clement Stone

I don't necessarily agree that we are completely the product of our environment. I do know it has a huge effect on our success in achieving the well-being we want and deserve. Health promotion advocates say that to achieve physical, mental and social well being, a person needs to be able to access personal and social resources to meet their needs, be able to identify and realize their aspirations and be able to cope with and improve the environment.

According to the Ottawa Charter for Health Promotion, "The fundamental conditions and resources for health are peace, shelter, education, food, income, a stable ecosystem, sustainable resources, social justice and equity. Improvement in health requires a secure foundation in these basic prerequisites".

So yes, the environment can affect our well-being in more ways than just the absence of toxicity, clean food and air. We have to look at our cultural attitudes of racism and sexism. We have to look at educational and mobility barriers for the elderly and disabled. We have to look at whether or not our wage systems, costs of housing and rent, as well as the costs of food, are affordable enough so everyone can have access to the basics.

We also have to look at the state of our justice and policing systems and how this affects the lives of those impacted, social justice in general and our belief in a fair and equitable society. We all know our social environment is in need of repair. We have heard the reports by the military, as to what is really happening in long term care homes. We have seen the over policing and the injustices committed against our black and indigenous people. The Black Lives Matter has brought to the forefront the long overdue need to rethink our policing methods.

I have also watched how the government's Maintenance Enforcement system ignores court orders and fails to secure and ensure single parents get the legal payments needed to feed their children. In Nova Scotia these parents, mostly women, make up the largest group of people facing increased poverty in Canada. In addition, our social assistance and welfare systems still allocate some of the lowest amounts of support in the country. The payment amounts fail to provide basic physical needs.

Is social activism linked to health and wellness? I don't know how we can separate the two. Protesting, bringing attention to a problem and formally taking a stand for change, in a constructive way, is really just a way to express compassion for others. Everyone in society benefits when we do our part to try and correct the injustices we see. It is also a positive and healthy way to channel anger and outrage when we witness or experience something that offends our sense of right and wrong.

This applies to society at large as well as our workplaces, social groups, our neighbourhoods, our families and even our intimate partnerships. Fairness and justice are core values we need to uphold and honour in all areas of our life. Peace, social justice and equity are three of the prerequisites to good health noted above. These are inseparable from and mutually dependent on truth, fairness and justice. The absence of truth (lies) are a thorn in the side of all other virtues. I will save that for another book.

*There really can be no peace without justice.
There can be no justice without truth. And there can
be no truth unless someone rises up to tell you the
truth.
- Louis Farrakhan*

Stop Injustice

Kids don't always play nicely. A little wrestling is OK but it always goes too far no matter how many times you say, "stop before someone gets hurt". It is a wonder that children survive childhood. When my children were young, I felt more like a referee than a mother. I am now discovering that if you have more than one pet, the dynamics between pets is similar to those between children.

Monster is my nine pound Miniature Pinscher and Bandit is my nine pound Siamese cat. Both are similar ages, approximately one year old. Just kids. When the pets are resting they cannot let peace and quiet reign for very long. Bandit lies close enough to stretch out her paw and touch Monster. Monster reacts by biting Bandit's tail. Bandit then tackles Monster by wrapping her paws around Monster's midsection and lying on top of her. The fight is on. Soon fur is flying accompanied by yelping and hissing.

On Sunday morning I was alerted to how adults don't always play nicely either. CTV news had a special report on workplace bullying. According to the Canada Safety Council, highly skilled employees are often the targets of bullying. Bullies who are insecure and lack social skills, feel threatened and take-out their targets using slander campaigns and strategic moves to render the target unproductive and unsuccessful.

Victims of workplace bullying suffer a wide range of stress related problems. When targets complain, they are often perceived as the problem. Targets of bullying are often forced to leave their jobs because they succumb to the effects of stress or are the recipients of a constructive discharge (a case fabricated to have them fired). Over time, the effects can be long term and tragic.

Techniques used by bullies include focusing on exposing the target's minute flaws or inventing errors in the target's work. Bullies focus on defaming the reputation of the target. The nasty stuff that is often mislabelled or dismissed as personality conflicts or politics is bullying. The intent is to have Canada's Bill C-451 amend the Canada Labour Standards Code to prevent workplace bullying. This Act is cited as the Workplace Psychological Harassment Prevention Act.

Bandit and Monster are learning to play nicely with the introduction of a deterrent. My third pet Trigger is a ten year old ninety pound Doberman. When he has had enough of the fighting, he breaks up the episode with loud barking and intimidation. Trigger wouldn't hurt the little guys but barks within a few inches of their ears and has a row of teeth more than half the length of their little bodies. Their heads must vibrate from the impact of the sound waves. Headaches and big teeth are great deterrents. I wonder if Bill C-451 will ever be implemented and a deterrent for us human adults?

This is not only a workplace issue but affects our children in the school system. We all watched bullying and knew someone who was a bully when growing up. Unfortunately some of those bullies did not grow up and landed in our workplaces and neighbourhoods. There is even bullying within our own circles of friends, in our communities and in our families.

Victims of workplace bullying suffer a wide range of stress related problems including headaches, stomach problems, depression, sleep disturbances. The effects can be long term and tragic eventually leading to suicidal and homicidal thoughts and actions.

We had a terrible and well know case of a lovely young woman whose sexual assault was made public on social media. She was incessantly bullied online and the police failed to do anything about it. She ended her life as a result. This is a heart wrenching scenario that is not an isolated incident.

Examples of bullying both in person and online includes spreading malicious rumours or gossip that are not true, excluding someone socially, deliberately trying to intimidate a person through threats or profanity, undermining or deliberately interfering with a person's work, livelihood, business or social connections and support systems, making offensive jokes in person, publicly, online or by email, intruding on a person's privacy by pestering, spying or stalking, constant, persistence and unfounded criticism, belittling a person's opinions and tampering with a person's personal belongings.

In the workplace, examples of bullying includes removing areas of responsibly without cause, constantly changing work guidelines, withholding necessary information or purposefully giving the wrong information, assigning unreasonable duties, workload or establishing impossible deadlines (ensuring the individual will fail), reducing workload to create a feeling of uselessness, blocking applications for training, leave or promotion and tampering with a person's work equipment and resources.

If we want to make our environment happy and healthy to live in, standing up to bullies is a good way to start. It helps to understand bullying for what it is and recognize it when it is happening. Bullying has many faces.

It occurs in many places and situations.
It is often not recognized as bullying
It hides behind supposed "acts of kindness" or
"just joking".
It pretends to be helpful or concerned.
It uses "good" deeds to cover evil intentions.
It is a terrible menacing action.
It is an impassioned, collective campaign.
It is the act of cowards.
That excludes, punishes, and humiliates its target.
It travels through the workplace like a virus.
It infects one person after another.
Until the victim is viewed as a terrible person,
With no redeeming qualities.
- SG Williams
...
Every thought, word and deed sends out ripples

Adopt Aromatherapy

Aromatherapy has been around for a long time. It is not part of TCM but is an aspect of Feng Shui used to improve the energy in the home. There is a lot of science to back up the healing properties of essential oils. These must be pure oils and the manufacturing process is important. I have been trying them out at home and in the clinic and am really happy with how peppermint oil reduces headaches; spruce needle oil helps with respiration and how lavender oil reduces stress, for example.

Fragrances can move us, bring back memories, improve memory, give us courage and change our mood to help us feel more positive, energized, happy, relaxed, aroused, sleepy or creative. Essential oils activate the olfactory system (sense of smell) to trigger the brain and affect mechanisms for mood or healing. When used therapeutically, aromatherapy is considered a form of alternative medicine.

Essential oils come from natural sources, mostly plants that are either cold pressed, distilled or extracted into a solvent. Quality is important and they must be pure if you want to gain therapeutic effects. Synthetic scents are not beneficial. They are expensive but you only need a few drops at a time. Make sure the oils are in a dark bottle that carries the Latin name, the common name, the supplier name, the country of origin, the organic stamp and any other additive or oils, if diluted.

Unlike chemical synthetic scents, essential oils do

not have negative side effects. They are very balanced. However safety is important. For topical application on the skin, dilute the oil in a carrier (another oil, cream), do not overuse one oil, don't ingest them, don't put them in your eyes and keep them away from children. Also look at any precautions on the bottle because some fruit based oils can increase sensitivities to light.

There are a number of oils that are exceptionally good for relieving anxiety, stress and depression. Bergamot is my first choice for depression, anxiety and nervous tension while lavender is my favourite aroma for calming and balancing emotional extremes. If you want to increase mental stamina and improve concentration, add basil or black pepper. To help you feel more grounded, less irritable or anxious, add fir, black spruce or marjoram. Fir and black spruce also help with respiratory issues. Marjoram can be sedating and also eases joint pain. Neroli and roman chamomile are very relaxing and can help with sleep. Neroli also inspires confidence and is an aphrodisiac.

To improve your outlook on the world, some of the oils can do this by balancing the emotions in addition to relieving stress. Cardamom and orange remind us of life's abundance and combat negative thinking. Lemon, clary sage, grapefruit, tangerine and jasmine are happy oils and are great revitalizers and stimulants. Elemi and spearmint are calming. Spikenard is very calming (sedating). Clary Sage is good for panic attacks but has estrogenic action. Tangerine and grapefruit are also good to enhance weight loss.

We feel stressed when there is too much to do, things are not going as expected or as planned, we are not doing what we want to do, or we don't know what we want. Depression, a gloomy outlook, overwhelming feelings of irritability, guilt, sadness, unworthiness or hopelessness can be more deep-seated, temporary or chronic. Many people suffer from stress, anxiety and depression. You are not alone.

Essential oils, acupuncture and herbal therapy can help but also be sure to reach out to someone, see an MD or talk to a therapist, especially if your condition affects and interferes with your daily life. Here are a couple of my favourite recipes that I use and provide in my clinic, that you can make yourself:

Peace: This is an inexpensive mix that helps you sleep and makes you feel happier and more optimistic. It smells great. Who doesn't like orange with a hint of spice. To a 15 ml bottle of pure sweet orange add 10 drops of sweet marjoram and 10 drops of petitgrain. All three oils have sedative properties so don't use it while driving.

Relief: This is a great mixture for relief from headaches, stomach upset and lung issues. It also helps boost immunity. Some use it for any head issues like vertigo. It smells nice and is a good multi purpose recipe. To any size bottle add equal amounts of eucalyptus, orange, peppermint, lemon and lavender.

... Science is now confirming... Essential oils have healing properties on both physical and emotional levels. Absorbed through the skin and via the olfactory-brain connection through inhalation, they have been considered among the most therapeutic and rejuvenating of all botanical extracts throughout the ages.
- Valerie Gennari Cooksley

Practice Feng Shui

We have lots of wind and water here on the Eastern Shore. We are blessed. In Chinese Wind Water translates to Feng Shui. This is an ancient practice of positioning homes and designing structures, to ensure good energy and proper flow of energy. Originally this was used in the placement of grave sites to bring prosperity to families by honouring their ancestors.

Have you ever walked to an area or been inside a home that just feels good. Sometimes you can't explain it. Lakes, ocean views, lush forests with rolling hills are a pleasant sight for most of us, unless you still have painful memories of raking those fall leaves. There is a reason for that. Living things create good vibrant energy and life force.

The practice of Feng Shui has evolved from different philosophies and schools and is believed to bring good fortune. Good luck depends on good people, good timing as well as good energy. I practice Feng Shui because feeling good about my surroundings is important to me and it fits with the Chinese medicine I practice.

As an acupuncturist and TCM practitioner, I help people balance the energy in their bodies to promote healing. However, external energy in our environment and in our relationships also affects our health. Have you ever felt depressed when your house gets cluttered and messy? This is because the energy gets stagnant and affects how we feel. It also reminds us there is a ton of work waiting for us and it drags us away from what we really want to do.

Ultimately we want to bring fresh air and lots of light into our homes. We want the good energy to come in and linger there with a nice flow throughout the house. Being clutter free is important as is the layout, design and decorating, placement of the house, and the geographic features of the land surrounding it.

If you are purchasing a new house, getting a Feng Shui reading could be beneficial. I recommend it. A house with land sloping upward behind it and sloping downwards in the front is good. Looking for lush vegetation and water in the front would be ideal. However, most of us are stuck with what we already have. Do not despair.

There are tons of ways to improve your energy and work with what you have. Getting rid of clutter is the first thing you need to do. The rest can be done with proper placement of furniture, accessories and colours. You do not need to spend lots of money. Below are some examples of what to do and what to look for.

The front of the house is deemed where the formal entrance is and where most of us have large windows and the living area. Having a house sitting with its back on a gentle slope is ideal with the slope behind the house a little higher. If you are in a residential area, a building behind you can act as that upward slope to offer a sense of protection. Small slopes or other buildings or trees, on either side of the house are also beneficial. The ideal positioning of a house geographically is when the landscape looks like the house sitting in an armchair.

If you find yourself facing a street coming towards you, at the end of a dead-end, T intersection or a corner lot, or if you have busy traffic along a straight stretch of a highway for example, you may want to buffer that with a small fence or hedge of trees. Being in close proximity to a hospital, church, fire station, cemetery, police station etc., may also present an overwhelming influx of energies, positive and negative, so you will want to buffer yourself from these, as well.

If you are at the top of a hill, on a steep incline, overlooking a cliff or right at the edge of the ocean, the view is great but it may be too much of a good thing. There is so much energy coming at you that you may have trouble sleeping. It is like always being on watch or sleeping with one eye open. As long as you can close the curtains and shut off the view or retreat from the view, you should find refuge.

Once you are inside your house, the walls are your mountains. There are nine areas of your house that reflect areas of your life. If you improve the energy in each of these areas, you can improve these specific aspects of your life: wealth, love, fame, family, creativity, health, wisdom or career.

The fixes to enhance each of these areas should fit your tastes and do not have to use accessories from Chinese culture. When I started, my husband was afraid I would Feng Shui him right out the door, with all his stuff sent to the workshop. That didn't happen, but I did organize his office area.

The centre of this house is the health and well-being area. This area correlates to the earth element and you want this area to be vibrant, healthy and grounded. Living green plants, with rounded, not sharp leaves, stone or pottery accents and colours with yellows or browns are good. Some recommend pictures of the earth, stars, sunrise, vegetables or fruit.

The other eight areas depend on what school of Feng Shui you adopt. Some schools use special compasses, stars, numerology etc. The modern methods divide up areas of your home using the front door as point zero. The older more traditional methods divide the nine areas of the house by compass direction.

Each area of the house has unique qualities and is believed to affect specific areas of your life. Readings can get complicated because each area has a specific relationship with the others. The key is to have good balance and good flow throughout the house. However if one area is weak, it can throw the balance off. It is easiest to just enhance all areas equally.

For example the area in the north, represents the element water. In the modern model this is also point zero and corresponds to the main formal entrance of your home. This is the area of career and success. In terms of health it affects kidney, bones, hair, ears and is about restoration, philosophy, fear and wisdom. To enhance this area, install a healthy plant, water fountain or something representing gentle or slow moving water. The colours for this area would include accessories in dark blue or black.

The opposite side of the house, south, is fire and affects fame, reputation and future wealth. It is about prosperity, joy, relationship and affects the heart, tongue, blood vessels and complexion. This area can be enhanced with a tall healthy plant (no dead or dried plants), objects representing recognition and fire, a light source (tall lamp) and red, orange, yellow or green accents. A red candle is good in this area.

The centre of the house represents earth, health, well-being, integrity, sympathy, self-care, the intellect and affects the spleen, muscles, mouth and lips. The north east and southwest areas are also earth elements and are also enhanced by accents in yellow, brown and beige earth tones. However the north east also represents the mountain and is about knowledge and wisdom. Books, items in deep blue or green and spiritual representations are also good. The south west is the love and relationship area. It affects fertility and is enhanced by pink, red, white and peach colours. Items representing marriage or union, photos of happy couples or items representing love are appropriate here.

In general, other things you need to look for are areas of clutter, sharp corners, ceiling beams or low sloping ceilings. These features can negatively affect the energy causing it to stagnate, become too sharp or oppressive. Steep stairs and long hallways can also cause the energy to speed up. These deterrents can be improved through placement of furniture, plants, use of mirrors, crystals and wind chimes, for example.

The bathroom is another area that needs attention. As mundane as this area might seem, the bathroom is worth mentioning because you want good energy to enter, linger and flow nicely through your home. A badly placed washroom, such as one close to the main entrance, can cause your good fortune to go directly down the toilet. I like to keep the door closed, the toilet lid down and a silk plant next to the toilet, shielding it from the door, no matter where the bathroom is located in the house. Making it as spa-like, enjoyable and pleasant as possible is good for this area.

The most important area for enhancing wealth and prosperity is in the southeast area of the home. This area is related to both wind and wood and the colour is green. It represents academics, achievements, creativity and morals. It is good to add healthy plants and flowing water, perhaps a water fountain, to keep prosperity moving towards you. You want things made of wood, accents of green or purple or vibrant artwork of trees or flowers.

The east also represents wood but instead of wind it is thunder. This is the area that influences family and is about planning, vision, courage and life direction. Green colours and wood items also enhance the energy in this area, but accents in blue are recommended because this area is supported by water. This is a good place to put happy pictures of family members. Improving this area can enhance family dynamics in a positive way.

The west and northwest areas are also about people. The west area is metal-lake while northwest is metal-heaven. The west is about creativity, children, self-worth, righteousness, letting go and grief. The northwest is about helpful people, spirits, authority and respect. Metal objects and the colours gold, silver and white benefit both areas, while I would add black accents to the northwest area. The west would be a great place to put children's artwork and the northwest would be a good place for religious pictures or pictures of people who have helped or inspired you.

In the end, you need to love the changes you make to your living space and it needs to be practical. The furniture should be spaced so there is a good flow without blocking movement or sight lines. The bed should have a good headboard, not directly facing a door or a mirror, or placed so your head is under a window, on the same wall as a toilet or where you can see a toilet. The desk in your office should not cause you to have your back to the door and be placed at the farthest point from the entry, with the seat facing towards the door. Of course you need a big enough space to do this.

It is not possible to do everything. Just change a little at a time, do what you can and have fun with it. It is about balance. Some say it is not good to make too many changes at once and over time I agree with this. It is best just to change one thing and then sit with it and see how it feels. If anything, just getting rid of the clutter will do wonders not only for the external energy affecting you but for your internal energy as well.

When we throw out the physical clutter, we clear our minds. When we throw out the mental clutter, we clear our souls.
- Gail Blanke

8 Check Your Internal State

Clear Spiritual Clutter

Do you ever find yourself drawn to a particular book on your bookshelf or at a bookstore? I came into the house the other night to find that the cats had knocked one of my books out of the bookshelf, and into the middle of the living room floor. I took this as a sign that perhaps there was something in this book I was supposed to read.

Today I finally opened the book. It was called, Clear your Clutter with Feng Shui, by Karen Kingston. I have lots of Feng Shui books and clearing your clutter is elementary step one. I didn't need help with this so I never bothered to read it. The first page I opened at chapter 21 had a little tick mark on it. It said:

Clearing Spiritual Clutter:...the whole of the book

*has been about this…(it) obscures our vision…
hinders us on our path. Each of us has a life
purpose…Clearing clutter in all forms allows our
original purpose…to re-surface…to clear the debris
that prevents us from connecting with our Higher
Self.*

I did a little speed-reading from the back towards the front until I got to some familiar ground. Not only is it important to keep your house tidy so good energy can circulate, we need to keep our bodies, our mind, our thoughts, our relationships, our consciences and our intentions tidy.

This book put a whole new meaning to spring cleaning. There was definitely a message there for me. Thank you to my kitties. This is what I learned:

- Adopting healthy eating habits that can give you that perfect bowel movement helps with physical clutter in our bodies.

- Writing to-do lists and tying up the loose ends of tasks gives us up-time, to focus on the important things and clears up mental clutter.

- Examining why everything in your home has ducks or cats on it, or why you can't throw out something you don't need or use, could help identify blockages, or unmet needs, to clear emotional clutter.

- Accepting others for who they are and stopping the judging, criticizing, worrying, gossiping and mental chatter that makes us unhappy, clears psychological clutter.

- Seeking relationships that uplift us and forgiving others, recovers the lost bits of our spirit, making us more complete and clears spiritual clutter.

- Expecting good things, being grateful and trusting we will be cared for, makes it so, by clearing clutter from our connection to the universe, higher power.

So as the snow melts, days start to get longer and you wear-out the pages on that seed catalogue, don't forget to plan for a little extra spring cleaning this year. Getting rid of the clutter in the closets and under the bed can facilitate that deeper decluttering we could all use.

Examine Your Emotions

Tonight I watched Extreme Makeover on TV. I like decorating shows and in this episode, a family in need was given a new home. How wonderful! Earlier I had been sitting out on the deck listening to loons and feeling peaceful and calm. Now that has changed. I cried my eyes out. I found myself feeling weepy and reflecting on more difficult times in my own past.

Emotional Intelligence (EQ) is a measure of the ability to manage our emotions in a way that produces beneficial behaviour and optimal choices in decision making. It consists of four abilities: identifying how others feel; using emotion to assist the thinking process; understanding the root cause of the emotion; and being able to manage the emotions.

Those with a high EQ know what they are feeling, have good emotional self-control, are able to think clearly when experiencing strong emotions. They are able to make decisions based on their hearts and not just their heads. This makes them better able to get in touch with their passions and find a path in life that is fulfilling.

Suppressing emotions makes it harder to find our life path. It can also make us sick. Our life force needs to be flowing appropriately for us to be healthy. Just as blockages in the flow of qi from trauma can cause pain, extremes in emotions affect the flow of qi causing qi and blood stagnation, heat, dampness and phlegm. These patterns can produce a long list of physiological imbalances and physical symptoms. For example:

- Anger and guilt causes liver qi to rise creating symptoms such as headaches, high blood pressure, reproductive issues, vision loss and other issues such as depression and insomnia.

- Worry and pensiveness knots the spleen and stomach qi, resulting in possible digestive issues, weak muscles, fatigue, easy bruising, bleeding, varicose veins and other issues.

- Sadness and grief dissolves lung qi. This weakens the lungs and our immunity and can bring on respiratory issues, skin conditions and make us more vulnerable to colds and flu.

- Shock and fear causes kidney qi to descend and dissolve. This along with overwork can cause weakened fertility, bladder problems, hearing loss, per-mature grey hair, sore knees and back.

- All emotions slow down the heart qi which houses the mind (cognition) and the Shen (ruler of the Spirit). This may create anxiety and mood swings between happy, sad with insomnia.

If you find yourself feeling strong emotions, get in touch with what you are feeling. Don't get busy so you don't have to think about it. Don't blame someone else for feeling the way you do. Often we only see the shadow of the cause of our emotional imbalance when we see it reflected in someone else. Use the emotion as a fishing line to see what else may be swimming around in the depths of your unconscious. Only you can allow yourself to feel the way you do.

Also our health can affect our emotions. The physical, spiritual and mental aspects of our being are all connected. When you don't eat, get enough sleep or suffer from acute or chronic disease combined with the need to take drugs, these things can have an affect on our emotional balance.

Our mind is just a tool and is not who we are. When we quiet our minds from the noise of our thoughts and emotions, when we feel our bodies connected to the earth and everything around us, when we connect to our interior self, sense the bigger picture and feel gratitude for what the universe brings us, it is then that we can know who we are. It is then that we can sense the things that inspire passion in us and are the guide moving us towards our true purpose.

Find Your Authenticity

Words are funny aren't they? The same word can mean different things to different people. Some words just sound peculiar. Take "spoon" for example. I caught my kids laughing about that word in the car the other day. "Spoooooooon" does sound odd. Where does that come from? Perhaps that is the sound we make when we try to speak with it still in our mouths.

Other words can sound more alarming that they actually are. I had been experiencing computer error messages such as "A Catastrophic Failure has Occurred!" or "You have committed a Fatal Error!". Yet the computer just keeps on working with no obvious consequences. I was waiting for the monitor to explode. Words do not always convey a true picture of the message it is trying to convey.

On the weekend, I watched Michael Moore's Bowling for Columbine. It wasn't until I watched Fahrenheit 911, that I realized that perhaps Bowling for Columbine was not about that noisy sport of bowling and that perhaps I might enjoy watching it. I know the movie has been out for a long while but wow! What a mind-expanding, controversial perspective on American and Canadian culture. What rock had I buried myself under when this movie first came out?

I needed to know more about Michael Moore. Who is this guy anyway? The DVD I rented included additional footage of comments about the movie from Michael. On the DVD, he talked about his Emmy

Award speech and justified his highly controversial, highly publicized comments by offering his conscience and his desire to live authentically as reasons for his actions.

OK, but what does he mean to live authentically, I wondered. Is this something that makes people stand out from the crowd, creates uprisings and polarizes people in a storm of controversy? It implies to me authenticity requires nerves of steel, courage, determination, brutal honesty, craziness and impending danger caused by a proliferation of enemies.

The dictionary defines Authentic as meaning "genuine, like the real or original, not counterfeit or copied, conforming to fact and therefore worthy of belief." I did a Google search and found a site that said, "Your Authentic Self: Living an Authentic Life. We will learn how to live more authentically and purposefully with the help of ten experts".

So living authentically must mean living on purpose not just by accident. OK, who lives by accident? Do they get out of bed each day and say to themselves, "OK I'm alive, now what?" Does it count if my purpose in life is to work hard and retire in the Cayman Islands? Maybe the size of the purpose is what matters. Maybe it has to be something big and important enough to change the world. There are lots of people in history who have done just that. I bet they lived authentically but just didn't know what it was called.

I am really starting to feel a huge amount of stress. This is really heavy stuff. Now I wished I had only watched Flight Plan with Jodie Foster instead of Bowling for Columbine. A simple action movie, with no deep meaning and no thinking required, would have been easier. Now I find myself reviewing and questioning my whole purpose in life and the reason for my existence. At this point in my life, on the world stage, the second tree from the left is fine with me until I figure out the rest.

Time to Wake Up

Signs of what is happening in the world with global unrest, the inability to know truth from lies and the pandemic, are all telling us it is time. It is time to awaken from the cold, hibernation, introspection and protectionism, and some aspects of fear, that represent the winter-water element in traditional medicine.

We need to prepare our hearts and souls for change. We need to begin or continue to question the norms, customs, expectations and beliefs that others impose on us. It is not easy to be who you really are. It is especially hard to break away from the constraints family and friends put on us, to be who they think we are, and should be.

We each have the power to change the world. We are not only inextricably connected to our physical environment as science outlines in quantum physics, but we are also one with the invisible consciousness of the universe. Therefore our thoughts and actions not only affect our own health but the well-being of others and how the future is manifested.

If we look at how young children cope, we can re-learn how to be present, take each moment as it comes, be and do what feels right in the moment. As long as we keep our hearts and minds free from bad thoughts and intentions, we can be assured that our actions and words will flow from the best intentions. As a human being, that is the best we can do.

As adults who are awake, many feel hated and

misunderstood. Some wonder if they were conceived on the wrong planet. You are the light that will guide the world and expose the darkness for what it is. You are needed now more than ever.

If you are struggling, a holistic approach will help. Physical blockages can cause emotional and spiritual blockages and vice versa. Pain, for example, can be simple trauma or a vast multi-layered issue. Taking care of one-self not only allows us to be freer, but our vibes will help heal those around us that we love, even when they don't want to hear our opinions or accept what we believe.

Be Hopeful

What is happening politically in some parts of North America is uncovering, in a big way, what is wrong in the world. For too long we have propped-up a world of false and superficial peace that denies the existence of the darkness. We have all collectively played a role in this.

The true face of humanity is not the beautiful picture we paint. Do we do this to possibly delude or absolve our consciences of the need for action? To bring about balance, we need to love and listen to the messengers who are expressing their pain. We need to allow the painful words to move us towards introspection of what is dark in us.

Like yin and yang, we are both dark and light and the two must be in balance. True peace cannot come until all things are reconciled. This applies to both our internal life and our exterior world. In darkness we are negative, paralyzed and asleep. In light we are positive, active and awake.

While darkness is growing, at its darkest hour, it will always flow back again towards increasing light. This is the nature of yin and yang. This is our guarantee of hope.

Laugh and Learn

I don't know what it is that I laugh about but I know I laugh every day. It has helped me focus on joy and makes me feel younger. Acting silly and laughing with someone you trust, builds a connection and it boosts immunity. It benefits your health greatly to laugh and it helps set up a point of view about life. Instead of darkness and pain, it helps to look for that silver lining.

My husband and I went to a comedy show on our first date. It was in the middle of the week and raining. There were only a few people in the audience. We could not avoid becoming the brunt of some of the jokes. Nobody was able to escape. My husband, in particular, was a target and it was good for me to see how he handled that. It is over a decade later and we have been laughing every day since.

My husband loves to make up his own jokes. He is also the first to laugh at them. Some of them are not very good but I laugh because he is laughing, sometimes so hard he can barely articulate the joke. I too have learned to develop some wit and will often misuse words or make a play on a word. I love to exaggerate to the extreme, to the point of being ridiculous to explore an important concept or idea. My husband applauds me, laughs and cheers me on. Our constant exploration of the lighter side has shaped the tone of our life together.

No matter what has happened to us over the years we have been armed with a positive attitude, comedy and the ability to look at the big picture. At one time the community we live in, was overdoing the road signs and rules. We just chuckled to ourselves and said we should put up our own sign, Private Sign Do Not Read. We didn't do that because not everyone has a sense of humour. However we did put up a large smiling happy face flag that waves in our parking pad. Now we have a colourful flag saying, "Another day in Paradise" reminding us of our beautiful community.

I also try to inject some levity into the world around me. I have put playful objects in the woods along my road and beside my driveway. My mother-in-law used to have a plastic pig, sheep and cow she would put out on her lawn every summer. After she passed away, these tacky items were headed for the garbage. Instead we rescued them and put them in our yard in memory of her. Children passing by love it. If they look closely they can also see Drucilla, my sleeping dragon, a bunny and a fairy.

Comedy allows you to expand your mind to new angles and possible ideas. It helps open you up to unlearning and relearning what you thought you knew. It is a great way to foster creativity and build a connection to others. It allows you to question everything, even things considered sacred. I believe it can not only reduce our stress and improve our health but also change people's attitudes and change society.

If we are to find our true selves and heal ourselves and others, being able to learn from our experiences is key. The invisible world around us is not always so obvious. The shadows lurking in our internal world can hide for a long time and cause us problems. Developing the ability to learn about ourselves and see the signs the universe gives us, is much easier if we are open to learning.

There is a problem with our ability to learn new things. I found a clue to this when I was reading about how people learn. When we learn, we often make assumptions about a situation we experience because we already think we know or are too polite to ask questions. We then draw conclusions about what we learned from that experience, based on those poorly researched assumptions.

When we make decisions based on incorrect assumptions, we don't actually learn anything new. We just reinforce what we already think we know. This endless cycle or loop keeps us spinning in the same thinking. I call it loopy thinking. You see it all the time when people use research they find on the internet to support what they already believe. We all do it.

In addition to loopy thinking, there is also conditioned thinking. This is when we have been programmed to react and see things in a specific way. These arc based on logical arguments built around how we think about what we experience. To combat loopy and conditioned thinking, we need to be active learners by listening to others, uncovering our assumptions and practising frequent learning. The first step is to expose our assumptions by determining the root causes of problems and examining the validity of the assumptions.

Comedy is a really fun way to do that. I will sit through hours of so-so stand up comedy patiently waiting for a really funny nugget. It is often about societal assumptions that we all take for granted but are so wrong. I love that about comedy. Plus just one good belly laugh, for me, is worth it. The endorphins will keep me feeling good for at least twenty four hours. Try it.

Oh by the way, if you see my husband and I out in our yard shovelling snow dressed in matching gorilla suits, you will know why. Others may just think we are crazy but we will be laughing at ourselves for hours. It is part of our health regime.

What we learn from experience depends upon the philosophy we bring to that experience.
- CS Lewis

...

At the height of laughter, the universe is flung into a kaleidoscope of new possibilities.
- Jean Houston

...

[Humanity] has unquestionably one really effective weapon—laughter. Power, money, persuasion, supplication, persecution—these can lift at a colossal humbug—push it a little—weaken it a little, century by century, but only laughter can blow it to rags and atoms at a blast. Against the assault of laughter nothing can stand.
-Mark Twain

Enjoy the Now

Just this morning I was woken up with a knocking sound on the wall. My big orange cat was pawing at the TV, bumping it against the wall and making the noise that tells me the food bowl is empty. He knows that signal gets me up in a big hurry.

Then as soon as I got up, my little dog was very keen on going outside right away to explore. I was immediately faced with a cool blast of fresh clean air to shake off the grogginess and noticed the wonderland of beautiful snow covered trees.

Ah! These little critters know how to bring you out of your head and your thoughts into the now. Because of my furry family members, my day now promises to be much more productive and I am able to enjoy the sun coming in the side window, that I would have missed, if I had slept longer.

Pets and children have a gift for bringing us back into the present and helping us to enjoy life's moments that we may have missed otherwise. This is important because the present is the only thing we can count on. There is nothing we can do about the past and even if we do everything right, there is no guarantee the future will unfold as planned. The present is all we have.

The present is the place where we make good memories, do good things, help others and engage in relationships. The present time is also the place where we care for ourselves, take care of our health and heal.

You may have taken good care of yourself in the past and plan to get back to taking better care of yourself in the future but only doing it now will do you any good.

People who are present and there for us, can have a profound impact on our lives. Over the years, I have met a few people who were really gifted in that regard. Even though our paths only crossed for a moment, there was a connection and somehow I was changed and made better by the encounter. I will never forget them.

The greatest gift we can give another person is a package of time in the present moment where we actively listen to, hear and see the other person, even if it is just conversation over a cup of tea.

So as we move into the New Year, my resolution is to be more aware that when the cats walk across my keyboard, I am the one who has strayed and it is time to take a break and enjoy the now.

9 Raise The Vibration

*"Concerning matter, we have been all wrong.
What we have called matter is energy, whose
vibration has been so lowered as to be perceptible to
the senses. There is no matter."*
- Albert Einstein

Everything is made up of particles that vibrate at various frequencies including rocks, plants, water, the air we breathe and every inanimate object we see. We exude energy and we absorb energy. Nothing is actually solid. Instead, objects are vibrating at frequencies that just make them appear solid. What we eat, what we do, what we think, what we feel and what surrounds us, is external energy that extends to, connects with and ultimately affects our internal energy.

If you look at the three states of water from ice to liquid to gas. What state water finds itself in, depends upon the amount of energy the water has. Warm up liquid water and supply the atoms with more energy, the electrons will start vibrating at a higher speed. Eventually, at its boiling point, the molecules have so much energy they fly apart. The water magically disappears as it changes from liquid to gas and disappears into the atmosphere.

The things we cannot see (like gases in our atmosphere) are vibrating at high frequencies. Our limited sense of sight doesn't let us see the movement, or vibration of the particles. We know they are there because we can do chromatography testing to detect them. Just like light which vibrates from low frequency (radio) waves to high frequency (gamma) waves, we can only see a small portion of the visible light as colours. I also wonder if the reason we can't see spiritual beings is because they are vibrating at higher frequencies.

Energy flows in a series of constantly oscillating wave forms. Frequency is measured by the height of the waves (base to peak) and how far apart they are spaced (peak to peak). The higher and closer together they are, the greater the magnitude of the frequency. Energy waves also "resonate" when they are smooth, regular and evenly spaced. This is what the natural form of energy looks like.

Resonance is also a common vibration where things move in unison so when something "resonates" with you, you understand and feel something in common with it. There must be a natural and healthy level of vibration and state of resonance for humans. Does it not make sense that our energy should be high and resonate (be smooth, regular and match nature), if we want to be healthy? If the waves are choppy and irregular, there is an issue and this is not-natural.

Every object, including human organs, have a natural healthy vibratory rate referred to as "resonance." If a part of the body begins to vibrate out of resonance or harmony, it creates what we term dis-ease.
- D. Takara Shelor

...

In 1992, Bruce Taino ... determined that the average frequency of a healthy human body during the day time is 62 to 68 MHz. When the frequency drops, the immune system is compromised.
- Susan Anderson

Bathe your Body in Good Qi

Just think about how good it feels to walk in the forest, along the beach and stand in the sun on a clear day. Sitting in the sun every day, just for a few moments can alleviate depression. Everyone loves to be next to the water and walk along the beach. Water holds and concentrates qi energy and we feel rejuvenated just by looking out the window at the trees and the water. This is nature increasing the vibration of our personal energy and healing us.

The only way to extend our lives, is to supplement the qi we were born with through the air we breathe and the food we eat. We conserve our life force by the way we live. Being in nature supplies high energy directly to our lungs especially when the air is clean. I believe salt air has a higher vibration because as a food, good natural salt has lots of minerals and is considered a high energy food.

Eating a traditional diet focused on natural, not processed, whole not modified, as well as fresh and local, ensures a good vibration in the food we eat. High energy foods are fresh and natural fruit, herbs, vegetables, spices, nuts and oils. Plants in particular have spent their lives converting the sun's rays, the air and the minerals of the earth from nothing into something pretty spectacular.

Being in tune with your body and the messages it is sending you helps you to adjust to a healthier lifestyle. One of the jobs as a holistic healer was the questioning at the beginning of each session. How was your sleep? Did you pee in the night, how many times? Were you awakened by dreams, what happened? Any pain, gas, burping after eating? What does your bowel movement look like? Any heart palpitations, hot flashes, unusual sweating, cough, shortness of breath, skin rashes? Do you have any pain, was it alleviated by pressure, by cold or by heat?

On and on I have many more questions. It is my job to know every detail so I can properly diagnose any pattern imbalance. The side effect of this is that every time my patient comes to see me, they know I will ask detailed questions. They start paying attention to every sign and symptom so they can report them to me. This is perfect for both of us.

We can all be our own detectives, investigating and interpreting our own body language. The more we pay attention to the body's messages and respond to them, the better we will be at alleviating the symptoms of disease before they become a problem. In fact we can probably prevent many diseases this way.

Once we feed ourselves energy, it is important that we try to conserve and concentrate that acquired post heaven qi. We can only digest well when we are happy, calm and thinking good thoughts. Qigong helps pull more energy from our surroundings. Then slow, deep breathing helps us make more efficient use of it. In this way we can maximize the food and air to give us the most nutrients.

According to Dr. Royal R. Rife, every disease has

a frequency. He found that certain frequencies can prevent the development of disease and that others would destroy disease. Substances with higher frequency will destroy diseases of a lower frequency. The study of frequencies raises an important question, concerning the frequencies of substances we eat, breathe and absorb. Many pollutants lower healthy frequency. Processed/canned food has a frequency of zero. Fresh produce has up to 15 Hz, dried herbs from 12 to 22 Hz and fresh herbs from 20 to 27 Hz.
- Susan Anderson

Elevate Your Mind Qi

If everything around us emits invisible waves that affect our energy, how can we protect ourselves? The people we surround ourselves with and the environment we find ourselves in, can either deplete us or energize us. Our mind can also trigger emotions that can cause us to feel upset or stressed. Therefore surrounding yourself with good people, fostering good thoughts, seeking calm and taking charge of your mind, is key.

So how do we control what goes in and out of our head? When we meditate, we become acutely aware of the problem of the numerous out-of-control thoughts. Where do all these thoughts come from? Some we don't even know are lurking in the background. When you wake from a lucid dream, it is always amazing how sometimes the dream seems to take on a life of its own and other times we can control the direction. Our mind is a mystery and it is a powerful tool. It affects everything in our lives including how we feel about ourselves.

Our mind is not who we are and we need to be aware that our mind is a tool we need to command. The mind can actually lead us astray if we are not careful and we believe everything it tells us. It is helpful to balance the mind's work by paying attention to the things we cannot understand like our body language, gut feel and intuition. The mind does not know everything.

Meditation is a good way to check in and pull back

the curtains of what is going on in the mind. The other gauge is our emotions. When we feel upset, we need to go back and comb through the thoughts that lead us there. Sometimes you will find a rogue idea that was planted there by an outside force. Like a long gone teacher saying, "you will never amount to anything". Perhaps a thought such as that has been planted and growing in the corners of your mind, hidden in the shadows. You may not believe the thought but sometimes these niggling little pests play with your subconscious self.

You may find yourself reacting emotionally in a way that is disproportionate to a particular situation. This is a clue that this is one of those nasty alien thoughts we need to work on. It is important to locate them and exterminate them. Fear in its many forms is one such invasive pest most of us have in the gardens of our minds. Finding it and uncovering its disguise is the first step. Replacing that fear-monger with a new thought, more logical reasoning and affirmations, can hold the healthier thought in place.

We must guard ourselves against people who consistently mess with our lovely mind-garden. Meditation, journaling and talk therapy with someone we trust, can help us keep a check on our mental health. We can also monitor what we watch on television, what books we read and what movies we watch. I know someone, you know who you are, who loves to read crime stories and watch the news, especially CNN. Then I see that they are feeling a bit depressed. All that gore, especially this pandemic news, has a profound effect on us.

This is one example of how I keep my mental health in check. I try to balance my need to know with how I am feeling about the content on the television. I will watch the news until I feel stress butterflies in my stomach. Then I switch to something cheerful. Anything with light comedy works for me. Last night however, I found myself laying on the couch with a video of Tibetan singing bowls ringing in the background. I knew I really needed it at this time. Some level of awareness about how I am feeling at all times is something I need. I believe we all need something similar, as part of a regular mental health regime.

Mindful meditation, journaling, positive affirmations and increasing our knowledge in the areas of energy healing, our own medical conditions, our symptoms (messages from our bodies) as well as using crystals, aromatherapy and colours, can help us take back and root out, any unhealthy wanderings of the mind.

Get Past the Ego

When we are overly mind centred, we can lose control over our mind's creations and give the ego free reign. The mind creates a false sense of who we are as unique, special, important and separate from others and nature. It ignores the idea that we are all connected and it needs input from the world around it to feed that separateness and sense of importance. Anything that threatens self importance is the enemy and it breeds conflict with what we truly feel. The ego is an artificial construct of the mind and its need to dominate makes us unhappy and casts a shadow over our authentic self.

Plus the ego is no fun at all. It is a real downer when it comes to an elevated vibrational state. It cannot laugh at itself. That is not healthy. We know that laughter is good for us. It is a great way to raise the frequency of our vibrations. However it is also not healthy to laugh at someone who has a big ego. Just the slightest incongruence with their belief in respect due and hierarchical position, will be aggressively challenged. For some narcissists attacking their ego is as serious as life and death.

I have seen people go to jail just because they laughed at a big ego. There is no limit to what a big ego will do to defend its own sense of self no matter how false it is. The ego is the great pretender and the one it fools is the person it rules. In the past I have always made an effort to protect myself from my own ego. I try to stay off that proverbial pedestal. If I don't climb up on it in the first place, I can't get knocked off. However, I know none of us is ego free. It is part of the human condition.

A few years ago I was bullied on social media. Terrible lies were said about me, publicly on my own Facebook page. I realized then that I still had an unhealthy ego that I needed to confront. I was embarrassed. I tried many ways to make it stop but before it did, I eventually found a way to laugh about it. I told myself that if you don't have haters, you are not doing enough. My haters are now a symbol that I am doing something right.

The many people in my community that know me, know the truth. I only care about the opinions of those who are part of my life and are important to me. The rest is noise that interferes with and depresses the good frequencies. It was a good reminder for me to keep my ego in check and re-subscribe to the idea that what other people say about me is none of my business. The main thing is that I do not let others affect how I feel about myself and lower my personal mind energy.

If you want to find the secrets of the universe, think in terms of energy, frequency and vibration...
"If you could eliminate certain outside frequencies that interfered in our bodies, we would have greater resistance toward disease.
- Nikola Tesla

Tap into Spirit

We have a spirit that can also detect issues and is sending us messages. That event you just have a gut feel about and really don't want to go to. Just don't go. Over time you will start to see the wisdom of your gut feel. Energy is the message sent by vibrational frequencies that communicates with us in profound ways. It allows us to sense things that we can't understand with our minds. It can tell our cells to heal themselves or cause us to affect and be affected by the energy beings around us.

Our heart also tells us what we need to do, where we need to go or who we need to be with. It is sometimes harder to understand. It is like the heart has another mind. I know that the gut has been labelled the second brain. I believe that it is the heart that is the seat of the soul. The heart houses the Shen, controls the Shen and is the emperor or ruler. That makes the heart the supreme brain, in my books.

Chinese Medicine considers Shen to be one of the three treasures that constitute life: Jing, the essence; Qi, the life force; and Shen, the spirit. TCM views the spirit as an integral part of our health and our well being and cultivation of the spirit is considered essential for health maintenance.

Chinese masters say it is through Shen that we radiate ourselves into the world. This spiritual radiance manifests as our wisdom, emotional well being, and ability to see all sides of an issue. Shen

This makes so much sense to what I have learned in my own life experience. Growing up I was always aware that the head and the heart would often be in conflict with one another. Our world puts great emphasis on the mind and believes it to be paramount to anything else. In fact doctors and scientists believe we only exist because of our minds. That is who we are. I do not believe this. My experience tells me it is our heart that connects us to spirit and rules who we are.

Age has taught me to always trust my heart first, even though my mind does not always understand the decision until much later. When I am heart centred, I am filled with inspiration, creativity and knowing. I know that my heart will always steer me in the right direction. I know that the universe loves me and I know that I am valued and respected. It is a great place from which to view the world. Connecting to the heart is a huge source of high frequency vibration. The more time we spend there, the healthier we become.

Being aware of our emotions helps us to keep our mind and heart in touch with spirit by removing obstacles that keep us from going there. Keeping our ego in check, forgiveness, releasing strong emotions, finding things to be grateful for, accepting difficulties as life-lessons and seeing others as your-other-self, builds compassion and connection to your heart. The connection to the heart is a connection to our spirit soul.

The heart is also the biggest energy centre of the body that grows when you think about the needs of others or are connected to your higher power, God or the universe. That heart energy radiates from your hands and allows you to heal yourself and others using visualizations and detailed directed intention. When supported by like minded others, such intention is powerful.

If we possess the spirit of the universe in every cell that is also connected to the universe that surrounds us, this is a connection we need to explore. This totality of good health is the solid foundation we need to build on, to better heal ourselves and others. The more we resonate with our true nature, others and the natural world around us, the more balanced we become.

But how do you connect to that spirit within you? Does it really exist? Where does it live?

The secret gateway to the spirit is gratitude. Some say this is the highest of all virtues. Others say it is thankfulness with a sense of wonder. Gratitude is something you can take action and control by the way you look at your life and the events in it. You can tune yourself into being grateful with your mind as a key. When gratitude is practised regularly, you will connect to that spirit, the energy of the universe and know that your soul is connected to all that is and resides in your heart.

Enjoy Sound

If we are connected to everything through energy, it makes sense that natural, healthy, external energy sources should be able to restore our internal imbalances. Sound healing is one of those modalities that is not only extremely enjoyable, but can push your choppy, wayward energy waves back into their natural, smooth and harmonic shape.

I use tuning forks, singing bowls and music tuned to nature in my clinic. I always had my water fountain on to simulate nature and sometimes I will even do some drumming. I always use my essential oils not only in a burner for the room but I select a specific oil and place it on a tissue on the chest for specific healing needs. These oils are known to have some of the highest vibrations in nature.

With the tuning forks, I use ohm for relaxation, a 528 Hz fork for healing and a very high pitched fork that clears negative energy and is believed to connect to angelic realms. I rake the healing fork through the patient's energetic field slowly from far away to close with the intention of helping them "bring in" any distant, past emotional disturbances that need to be retrieved and processed.

I use Tibetan singing bowls that I sounded out to a particular scale, that resonates with the energy centres of the body (the chakras). I play each one from root to crown hoping to leave the patient vibrating in the crown chakra while getting the needles, so that they can get extra help with the healing.

After the needles are in, I play music that vibrates at the right frequency and has a positive effect on the body. From my studies certain music is more effective at this than others, because of specific frequency blueprints, I use music tuned at 432 Hz or use the Solfeggio scale. The frequencies of this ancient scale, first used in Gregorian Chants, are divisible by the numbers 3, 6 and 9 and are in tune with nature from a mathematical perspective.

I always hope that my clients can enter a meditative state while letting the needles work. Drumming can certainly help with that too. I usually use that in a group circle and have really enjoyed drum circles. There is nothing that is as powerful as being surrounded by a group of drummers, drumming with the intention to heal self, others and the community. The patterns of sound that naturally emerge are often beautiful. You can feel the vibration of the circle dramatically increase.

In the beginning, I only used the sounds for those I felt would be open to it. However I found it hugely beneficial and I created a little regime of healing vibrations and made it part of every treatment. I do not always explain why I am doing it, other than to say "I am just getting the wrinkles out of your energy".

If parts of the body become imbalanced, they may be healed through projecting the proper and correct frequencies back into the body.

- Jonathan Goldman, Healing Sounds: The Power of Harmonics

Feel the Qi

You can use your hands or finger tips to tap on acupuncture points or whole meridians to raise the vibration of your body. You do not need needles for these points although the needle is the most powerful way to use them. Points along your eyebrows and on your cheek bones or the top of your head can provide stimulation for the senses, open the orifices and "pull up" your qi. You can look up the Emotional Freedom Technique (EFT for example) that uses many of these points.

You can also use your fingers to locate, press and hold the points. This is called acupressure. The points are named after the meridian on which they are located followed by a number. These points have tons of good actions on the body. You can look these up.

Some that I like include:
   Du20, Du24,
   Gallbladder(Gb)20, Gb21,
   Kidney(Ki)27,
   Ren12,
   Small Intestine(Si)3,
   Triple-Warmer(Tw)5, Tw6,
   Pericardium(Pc)6,
   Stomach(St)36,
   Gallbladder(Gb)34,
   Spleen(Sp)6,
   Kidney(Ki)3
   and Liver(Lv)3.

Qigong, as described earlier, is a great way to raise

your vibration. Before I start I like to swing my arms from front to back while hitting the area below my navel and then my lower back, repeatedly. This wakes up the core energy centre for the body. The qigong movements open any blockages and get the qi flowing. Then at the end, rising on your toes and plunking yourself down on your heels, sends vibrations throughout the body for a final shake up.

Using your voice and chanting is also effective. In qigong there are sounds for every organ system. You can, however, just make whatever sounds you want and feel the humming vibration move to different areas. One good routine is to visualize an energy ball over the three energy centres of the body (at the base of the skull to the third eye, in the centre of the chest and just below the navel and into the lower back).

At the same time of the visualization at each centre, vocalize sounds for each area (Weng for head, Ar for heart area and Hong for the lower abdomen). Place your hands with fingers touching and palms facing toward the body in front of each energy centre at the same time as the chanting and visualization. It is important for the palms to face the body, not away from the body to direct the energy from your heart to your hands inward. Being grateful activates the heart, so finish each centre by repeating thank you.

The laying on of hands is an old Christian concept that invoked the higher powers to spontaneously heal someone when the hands were placed on the body. Many people use similar techniques using Reiki for example. I believe that my hands are a source of healing energy. It is one of the energy centres of the body.

I had heard that Therapeutic Touch® was being used in our local hospitals. This modality has been greatly studied and has accumulated a lot of scientific evidence to support its efficacy. So I chose to adopt this and learned to channel the energy in my hands using this technique. There is no actual touching and the hands just hover close to the body. I found this practice works well with my acupuncture. The teachers are wonderful and wise and their support is amazing.

The energy another person emits, communicates with our energy. With practice you can get signals from the field to tell you what to do, if you are well grounded, focused and compassionate. Signals can take many forms but a simple example is, if you feel a cold area, you would direct, through intention and visualization, a warming light to balance that area. After sweeping, evaluating and balancing the entire field, with hands 6 to 12 inches away from the body, the person should experience increased relaxation, calm and well-being.

Supercharge Intention

One of the first things I learned at acupuncture school was to set my intention at the tip of the needle. What does that mean? I knew it was a profound statement but it would be years before I realized just how much. Whole books have been written about how important intention is. Then as I learned Therapeutic Touch®, I experienced how intention combined with compassion was key.

I have read from Wayne Dyer, that if you are connected to the power of intention, you radiate energy that affects everyone around you, like ripples in a pond. When you see that your intention brings about your desires, your belief in its abundance grows and creates a fountain of power. You start to manifest your world by co-creating it with intention.

Staying focused on a detailed intention can be difficult. Healers like Adam McLeod (Dreamhealer) have fine tuned this to an art and have taught many people how to do this. Adam says to get as much detailed medical information as possible and for at least 20 minutes in the morning and at night, picture the person that needs healing in a 3D hologram type of image. Watch as little lights or a waterfall or sparks take over the diseased area and replace the area with healthy tissue. You can use whatever visuals you need to stay with the healing process.

In Theta Healing, there is another form of visualization. You see yourself move out of your body and up through your chakras into a space continuum where there is all knowing and no time. You keep going up and beyond to the white light. You state the healing that will happen. Then you come back down into the person in need of healing. Watch the healing take place as you thank the universe that the healing is done. The key here is that you ask and see that it is fulfilled, right there and then. No hoping for it to happen in the future. It is done.

The intention of a healer is to always help, not harm. Always to be open and caring. Intention is powerful. It is more than that however. After a decade of using my skills to help people heal, I found that compassion is equally as important. A mentor, I highly respect, told a class of graduating acupuncturists, "The most important thing you can do is to love your patients. They will know if you love them or not".

Love is actioned through compassion. You can't really help people heal, if you are not compassionate. You can't be compassionate if you don't love. You can't love them if you judge them and don't see them as they really are. I had the privilege of hearing the stories of struggle, triumph and defeat and seeing strength and beauty in each client. I was often in awe and I believe this is a reflection of how the angels see us.

We are all heroes, heroines and warriors, each in his and her own right. As my husband says, we are all the number one stars in our own life. If you do really listen, and see others, the dynamic of healer and patient together opens up a shared energy field. Here is where spirit allies come in and commune with you. It is a powerful experience where high level frequencies are supercharged. Each person comes away with new insights and inspiration.

To be in balance everyday and not take on the woes of your patients, takes a dedicated spiritual practice. Some call it grounding but however you do it, you need to connect to the earth's energy, the spirit within you and the omnipresent spirit that surrounds you. By practising the art of gratitude every day this becomes easier over time. It also makes life so much more enjoyable when you see the world through a thankful window.

It is in that mix, that a healer experiences intention fuelled by compassion, supported by spirit through the gateway of gratitude. This is really a three legged stool that supports our words and the detailed vision of what we want to create for ourselves and others. When you add prayer, which I do, this is the stuff of miracles. The result of this combination creates a high frequency healing bubble filled with, what I call, supercharged intention.

The power of intention is the power to manifest, to create, to live a life of unlimited abundance, and to attract into your life the right people at the right moments.
- Wayne Dyer

...

The highest intention comes from love and compassion ... when our intentions come from a place

of love and compassion then we have the power of the universe... Intentions compressed into words enfold magical power.
- Deepak Chopra

...

In the universe there is an immeasurable, indescribable force which shamans call intent, and absolutely everything that exists in the entire cosmos is attached to intent by a connecting link.
- Carlos Castaneda

10 SEEK TO HEAL & BE HEALED

It does not take a special person to believe in miracles and make them happen. Healing is about becoming whole, balanced and being your true self in the world. It is a hard thing to do when how we perceive ourselves is so biased by the social norms and culture of the people around us. Society tells us how to behave, what roles to play and what or whom should be considered valuable.

The most devastating disease in the world today, I believe, is the attack on self esteem and the manifestation of self-hate. We are constantly being told and reminded that we are never enough. The magazines show people always well dressed in beautiful homes. Movies and television, even when trying to display real life, do not. Neither does our Facebook feeds where we pose as our glamorous selves and post a fantasy world. It's hard not to compare ourselves to others.

The world has become increasingly narcissistic. People are more and more selfish and the culture is a belief in scarcity not abundance. We clamour to get ahead of others and take from others. People are not always kind, some spread hate and some bully others to make us feel smaller to combat their own issues with self worth. This perpetuates this disease and a pandemic of self-loathing.

I want to say that many of us have been so deeply hurt and injured, that the thought of being healthy and healed seems impossible. Healing is not easy. As I try to simplify the process and tools to heal, I want to acknowledge that some pits are so dark, professional help and support is a must.

We have all suffered trauma in some way. As individuals we are all impacted differently, some more severely than others. Many have lost their way, given in to the belief that they are not valuable and have resorted to self harming behaviours. Please seek help. You are a valuable soul and worth it.

Many of the best healers are those who have come out of a dark place and survived. Some call it the dark night of the soul. How else can a healer help someone surrounded in darkness if they have never been there or know the place and landscape. If you are such a person suffering, know that the deeper the pain etches into your soul, the greater joy you will be able to contain and the greater compassion you will feel for others, once you get to the other side.

Compassion is not a relationship between the healer and the wounded. It's a relationship between equals. Only when we know our own darkness well can we be present with the darkness of others. Compassion becomes real when we recognize our shared humanity.

- Pema Chodron

...

Compassion asks us to go where it hurts, to enter into the places of pain, to share in brokenness, fear, confusion, and anguish. Compassion challenges us to cry out with those in misery, to mourn with those who are lonely, to weep with those in tears. Compassion requires us to be weak with the weak, vulnerable with the vulnerable, and powerless with the powerless. Compassion means full immersion in the condition of being human.

-Henri Nouwens

We were born into this world to be happy, fulfilled, to help others and to coexist peacefully with one another. Every person who takes on the work of healing and achieves it, sends ripples out into the world that helps heal others. The quest is worth it and to save our world each of us can do our part. It starts by knowing that the powers that created us and that continue to love us, knows us best and sees our value. Every person is a shining star that even the angels revere. Please know that you are loved even though it seems that this world hates you.

The universe does send us reminders of this love even in our darkest hours. It could be a bird that comes to the window, a rainbow or just the kind smile of a stranger walking by. If the power of creation cares for every little bird, animal and insect, then how can we doubt our worth? We just have to ask and watch how we too are cared for. Everything in our lives happens for a reason, for our own personal growth, as terrible as that may seem. There is always a silver lining. Help is there at every turn if we ask.

I love this poem called If by Rudyard Kipling. I just overlooked the last line. I think this is for everyone because life can be just like this:

If you can keep your head when all about you
Are losing theirs and blaming it on you,
If you can trust yourself when all men doubt you,
But make allowance for their doubting too;
If you can wait and not be tired by waiting,
Or being lied about, don't deal in lies,
Or being hated, don't give way to hating,
And yet don't look too good, nor talk too wise:

If you can dream,
and not make dreams your master;
If you can think,
and not make thoughts your aim;
If you can meet with Triumph and Disaster
And treat those two imposters just the same;
If you can bear to hear the truth you've spoken
Twisted by knaves to make a trap for fools,

Or watch the things you gave your life to, broken,
And stoop and build 'em up with worn-out tools:

If you can make one heap of all your winnings
And risk it on one turn of pitch-and-toss,
And lose, and start again at your beginnings
And never breathe a word about your loss;
If you can force your heart and nerve and sinew
To serve your turn long after they are gone,
And so hold on when there is nothing in you
Except the Will which says to them: 'Hold on!'

If you can talk with crowds and keep your virtue,
Or walk with Kings nor lose the common touch,
If neither foes nor loving friends can hurt you,
If all men count with you, but none too much;
If you can fill the unforgiving minute
With sixty seconds' worth of distance run,
Yours is the Earth and everything that's in it,
And—which is more—you'll be a Man, my son!

If we can get beyond self-hate and begin to believe we are worthy. If we can see a tiny bit of light shining from beyond that pit and just hold on. The way to healing is not beyond our reach. I do not believe that we were placed on this earth without the tools to thrive. When you boil down most of the healing theories and teachings of all healers, the base message is the same. At the core is one basic tenet or code, they all facilitate the raising of your personal vibration.

Raising your energy and the vibration is key.

Resonance is a common vibration where things move in unison so when something "resonates" with you, you understand and feel something in common with it. The more we resonate with our true nature, others and the natural world around us the more balanced we become.

Energy is the message sent by vibrational frequencies that communicates with us in profound ways. Knowing you are spirit expressed in a human body form, helps us to stay in touch with our soul self. That soul is your core energetic life force. It allows us to sense things that we can't understand with our minds. It can tell our cells to heal themselves or cause us to affect and be affected by the energy beings around us.

Being balanced means that we can move in the world without being overwhelmed by everyday events. Our health is maintainable and our body responds to our self-care. Emotionally we can process what happens in a reasonable manner and react appropriately. Energetically we feel connected to others and those we love. I call this the horizontal energy connection.

Being grounded means that we have our feet firmly planted on the earth. We are fully present in the now and focused on that conduit of energy that both connects us to the earth and connects us to heaven or a spirit plane. It is being in the middle place where we are not carried away to the past, the future or that spiritual place. I often visualize myself as a tree with my feet as roots and my arms as branches reaching upward. I call this the vertical energy connection.

When we are both balanced and grounded, we feel a sense of calm and a sense of optimism. We experience serendipity and see events magically unfold in a way that supports us and reminds us we are not alone. We feel we have a mastery over our lives like a surfer nailing the ride on a crest of a wave. I call this being in the zone.

When we are "in the zone" we are protecting and optimizing our health, our vibration resonates with nature and the creator-spirit, we are able to increase the qi of our bodies, minds and spirits and get the wrinkles out of our own energy bodies. On this good solid foundation, we know we are loved and lovable, we radiate good energy vibrations wherever we go. We cause others to feel hope, happiness, optimism and belief in something greater than themselves. We can spread love to others.

When surrounded by caring supportive people, learning, being conscious of our mind's activities, moving through the world as a healthy, high frequency individual, being true to yourself and seeking our soul self, we are capable of healing those around us. Our reach goes beyond time and space as those who are positively impacted by us, pay it forward. As they heal and vibrate at a higher level, they touch those in their lives. The good intentions we begin can create ripples that can heal the world. This is the code to empower healing and the way you do that is your own path.

*It is our purpose and destiny to live in conscious
oneness with our world, be present and know that our
true identity is in the reflection of the divine.*

*When your non-persona can tap into your passion
and your actions are directed by love, inspiration and
enthusiasm, your work will resonate in alignment
with the goals of the universe.*

*This is the secret to knowing your life purpose. A
purpose that you can fulfill every day you have the
courage to be true to what you know and what is
right.*

*In this way you will change the world with more
power than any one person could ever imagine or
accomplish.*
- SG Williams

Find Your Tribe

Believe it or not there are people out there just like you. No matter how weird you think you or your beliefs are. You are not alone and when you think you are, the universe will send someone to walk along your path with you, even if for just a little while. Some of us go through life thinking we were either born into the wrong family, born in the wrong century or for some, we think we may have landed on the wrong planet.

It takes time to learn what a good relationship looks like. Some of us are lucky enough to see it first hand with role models. Most of us learn by trial and error as we experience what it feels like to be around people that help us feel at peace with ourselves or not. We feel at peace when we are accepted for who we are by both others and ourselves.

Even better is to find someone who is interested in us and cares enough to actually listen and hear what we are saying. These valuable friends want to know the real you, not make assumptions about who they think you are. Often you can feel a connection with the people who get-you. You are not a role in a play on the stage planet earth. Don't be afraid to venture out beyond your known circle if you find yourself stuck with the wrong friends.

Good friends are those you can trust with your feelings and who are willing to reciprocate. They are the folks you can go to when times are difficult and feel safe. They are the folks that will not abandon you when you make mistakes or have a difference of opinion. Even if you can find one such person with whom you can experience just some of these attributes, this is priceless.

That resonance of energy with like minded folks gives you a sense of belonging and that you matter. Good relationships help you to see yourself in a better light through the eyes of those who love you and respect you. You can feel with your heart energy, who and what is right for you, when you practice paying attention to it. Your tribe will help you increase your energy and accelerate your own healing.

Healing takes love, compassion, intention, some divine help and friends. Some of us have spent a major part of our lives searching for this. Don't stop. This world needs healing right now. There are lots of folks out there, with the stuff needed to make that happen. I know because I have been privileged to meet so many of these folks in my healing practice. There are many of you good souls out there being that pebble, spreading ripples of healing energy. This book was written for you.

The highest degree of a medicine is Love.
- Paracelsus

Blessings from Me::

We were created to be healthy & happy.
Like the earth we undergo
a cycle of transformation
That is beautiful and perfect.
Awaken to this rebirth and be in awe
of the magic of each moment.
Feel the peace of gratitude envelop you.
See your true self in the reflection
of the still waters of your soul.
Know that you are perfect just as you are,
wonderfully made and worthy of love.
Specially created and unique.
Accept the care and respect and know you are
deserving of your rightful place.
- SG Williams

ABOUT THE AUTHOR

SG Williams is a qualified holistic alternative health specialist with a strong background in science and research. She has positively contributed to her own learning and her community for over five decades where she raised her three children. In the last decade she has successfully operated her own healing clinic.

For over more than three decades she has been involved in healthcare in some way. Her years in holistic health, included teaching, health promotion and caring for seniors in addition to being an acupuncturist. Since 2008, she has acquired the skills and experience to successfully treat patients with a wide range of complex issues encompassing mental, emotional, spiritual and physical well-being.

Ms. Williams has helped hundreds feel better, more balanced and more like their true selves. Her hope for everyone is for them to be able to experience their heart's discovery of health and happiness by being in the world, the way they were meant to be. She believes that this is what true healing is all about.